The Elements Of Cancer Survivorship

A Guide to Navigating the Journey

Dr. Crystal A. Champion

and

Marcia D. Dupree

Contents

Foreword 1
An Introduction To Cancer Survivorship 2
Section 1: The Diagnosis 4
Section 2: Financial Considerations 12
Section 3: Support And Advocacy 18
Section 4: The Power Of Hope 21
Champions Can! Foundation for Cancer Wellness, Inc. 30

The Elements Of Cancer Survivorship

Foreword

DISCLAIMER:

This guide was created to be a supportive resource for those who have already received a cancer diagnosis and is not intended to be a guide as to how to avoid, prevent, detect, treat, or cure the initial presence of cancer.

The aim of this guide is to stress the need for cancer patients to become their own advocates, armed with information that will help to minimize the fear, confusion, frustration and feelings of helplessness and disruption that invariably accompany a cancer diagnosis, it's treatment, and the general life changes that they bring. This body of work is also dedicated to those individuals who have had a personal journey with cancer or who have had friends and loved-ones who have been affected by this disease as well as those who are passionate about LIFE! May God grant you grace, peace, faith, hope, endurance, and healing.

An Introduction To Cancer Survivorship

The National Cancer Institute states the following in regards to cancer survivorship:

"Cancer survivorship focuses on the health and life of a person with cancer post treatment until the end of life. It covers the physical, psychosocial, and economic issues of cancer, beyond the diagnosis and treatment phases. Survivorship includes issues related to the ability to get health care and follow-up treatment, late effects of treatment, second cancers, and quality of life. Family members, friends, and caregivers are also considered part of the survivorship experience." So what exactly defines a cancer survivor?

A person who has had cancer is commonly referred to as a cancer survivor. A "co-survivor" can be used to describe a person who has cared for a loved one with cancer. Not every person who has had cancer likes the word "survivor" due to various reasons. This could be attributed to the fact that they simply identify themselves more with being "a person who has had cancer" or someone who is "living with cancer" and trying to manage it on a day-to-day basis. These reasons can cause a person not to think of themselves as a cancer survivor.

Living with cancer or a history of cancer is different for every person; however, most people have the common belief and expectation that life is different after cancer and the associated treatments.

Other common reactions that people have after cancer include:

- A better appreciation for life.
- Being more accepting of themselves.
- Feeling more anxious about their health.

- Difficulty or not knowing how to cope after treatment ends.

Cancer survivorship can mean the following:

- Having no signs of cancer after finishing treatment.
- Living with, through, and beyond cancer.

There are 3 phases of cancer survivorship:

Acute survivorship: Begins at diagnosis and goes through to the end of initial treatment. Cancer treatment is the focus in this phase (surgery, chemotherapy, radiation, etc.). Cancer survivorship actually starts at the time of diagnosis. It is at this time that individuals should impart themselves with as much knowledge as possible regarding their diagnosis in order to have a more favorable outcome and outlook, in addition to equipping themselves with the necessary tools needed to "survive".

Extended survivorship: Begins at the end of initial treatment and goes through the months after cancer treatment has ended. Interventions for the side-effects of cancer treatment are the main focus.

Permanent survivorship: In this phase, it has been years since a person has completed their cancer treatment. The chance of cancer recurrence is less and long-term effects of cancer and treatment are the focus of this phase.

The following sections will highlight how you should enter into and navigate through the 3 phases of cancer survivorship while learning how to navigate your cancer journey. The goal is for you to feel empowered and well educated regarding your cancer diagnosis, treatment, and after-care. Remember, **CANCER SURVIVORSHIP BEGINS AT TIME OF DIAGNOSIS!**

Section 1: The Diagnosis

So you have heard the dreaded words that you have cancer and have received an official diagnosis. Many varying emotions are a natural outgrowth ranging from shock, disbelief, and fear; to wishing and hoping that it would just go away; or downright denial that the diagnosis could be accurate. However, in the midst of this avalanche of emotions, it is incumbent upon you to begin the process of education, involvement and most of all, determination that you will not leave the future of your health solely to the medical professionals as you go through the healthcare process.

Key factors:

___You must know precisely the type, present stage and condition of the cancer, organs/systems that have been affected or have the potential to be impacted, and the anticipated recovery prognosis. **DO NOT BE <u>AFRAID TO ASK QUESTIONS UNTIL YOU UNDERSTAND!</u>** A good idea would be to have a family member or trusted friend with you while discussing the diagnosis with the doctor. You may be feeling overwhelmed and the other person can catch information stated that you either did not hear or forgot. Having a notebook along with you is a very good idea and ask your companion to make notes for you.

___Advise your doctor that you would like a second opinion, or even a third opinion if you feel that it is needed for you to be well informed about your condition. All too often patients are afraid to do this, but it is in your best interest to arm yourself with more than one doctor's input and insight. It is not uncommon for a doctor to have overlooked or misdiagnosed something.

___Do not allow yourself, a friend, or a family member to be rushed through the process of educating yourself as much as you can regarding your diagnosis. Make sure that you are well informed and feel confident about your treatment process before making decisions. With a diagnosis of cancer, it is very common

The Elements Of Cancer Survivorship

and appropriate to feel that you want to have medical intervention/treatment for your condition as quickly as possible so that you can get back to a healthy life. It is imperative that you have a clear understanding of all aspects of your treatment and care before proceeding. Through the process, keep in mind that **THIS IS YOUR LIFE AND HEALTH AT STAKE!**

If not proactively stated by the doctor(s), ask the following questions:

___What will the treatment plan consist of? (i.e. chemotherapy, radiation, targeted therapy, surgery, etc.?)

___How long will the treatment plan continue?

___What will be the frequency of the treatment(s)?

___How essential is it for me to keep to the treatment schedule?

___Can I postpone a session?

___What is the goal of the treatment(s)?

___What is the success rate of the proposed treatment that I will have? What are the chances of recurrence?

___If I need surgery, what are the different surgical procedures related to my condition and what option is best for my treatment?

___How will the treatment(s) be administered (i.e. intravenously via a port or vein, injections, creams, liquids, oral medication, topical, etc.?)

___If chemotherapy is the recommended treatment, could I have a port implanted? (A port is a small device imbedded in the body. Needles are inserted more easily through a port than directly through the skin.)

The Elements Of Cancer Survivorship

___Where will the treatment(s) take place (i.e. your doctor's office, a specialty clinic, hospital, etc.?)

___How many sessions of chemotherapy and/or radiation will be require if needed?

___How long does each treatment session last?

___What is my expected recovery time?

___Who will administer the treatment(s) (i.e. your doctor, specialty nurses, specialty technicians, etc.?)

___Will I be referred to a physician and/or oncologist who specializes in my specific type of cancer?

___What other medical professionals should I expect to see during this process?

___How should I dress in order to receive treatment?

___What are the names of each medication that will be administered?

___What is the dosage amount of each medication that will be administered?

___What specifically does each medication contain?

___How does each medication work in treating my type of cancer?

___What if I can't afford my treatments? What are my options?

___Are there any prescription drug programs that can offer assistance for my recommended medications? Can you request a cheaper drug or alternative on my behalf so that it is more affordable for me?

___Will I need to change my diet and if so, what will that consist of?

___How can I be as healthy as possible before, during, and after my treatment?

___How will I feel after each treatment?

___Are there other alternative, natural, or holistic treatments available for my diagnosis?

___What are the possible side effects?

___How can I diminish the side effects?

___How long could the treatment side-effects last?

___What symptoms or side-effects should I report to my medical care team?

___Will the treatment put at me at risk for developing another type of cancer or a secondary cancer?

___Are there any new developments or current research being conducted for the treatment of my type of cancer?

___Are there any clinical trials available for my specific type of cancer?

___How will the treatments affect my work and/or social life?

___How will my intimate life or the way I view intimacy and/or sex be affected?

___Will I have issues with my self-esteem/self-image?

___Will I lose my hair? If so, would that entail full body hair loss (i.e. cranial hair, eyebrows, eyelashes in addition to any other body hair? Would any hair loss be permanent? Is there anything I can do proactively or as a preventative measure to slow or prevent hair loss? (i.e. cold caps and cold therapy)

___Will I be able to work? If not, will my physician be able to provide me with the documentation necessary to extend time missed from work if needed?

___Will I feel better when the treatment(s) is over? How long will it take?

___What can I do to reduce the risk of my cancer recurrence?

___What long-term health issues can I expect as a result of my cancer and its treatment?

___What happens if there is an interruption in my treatment or care?

___Does the physician's office have a website/patient portal? If so, how is it accessed? What personal information regarding my account will I have access to view? How can I request copies of my medical records?

___During the treatment process, will there be other tests/procedures that will be required? If so, what could they consist of (i.e. blood work, scans such as EKG, CAT, MRI, outpatient surgery, etc.?)

___Does the cancer center or hospital provide counseling services?

___Is there a cancer survivorship care-plan available to me to support me through my journey?

___Can I continue my usual sports, hobbies, exercise regimen and other physical activities? If that is not feasible during treatment, can I take up my usual activities when treatment is complete?

___What if I have trouble with transportation to get to my appointments and treatments? Are there any resources available to me to help me with transportation needs?

The Elements Of Cancer Survivorship

Note: These are questions that you should consider asking your doctor and may not be an all inclusive list specific to your diagnosis or your lifestyle.

You should also request a printout listing the known side-effects of the treatment(s) you may have. Also document and keep a record of the side-effects (both physical and emotional) that you experience during your treatment and report them to your medical team so that your treatment may be adjusted, and other support tools can be recommended if needed.

Depending upon the specific type of treatment you will be undergoing, the medical staff with whom cancer patients interact can vary greatly. Here are some of the various personnel that may be encountered:

Medical Oncologist: Will oversee your overall cancer care

Radiation Oncologist: Will develop your treatment plan for radiation if you must undergo this treatment

Surgical Oncologist: Will address cancer treatment and/or removal through surgical procedures

Oncology Nurse: Will care for you if you are admitted as an inpatient to the hospital during your course of cancer treatment. Will also administer chemotherapy IV infusions at cancer treatment centers or clinics

Oncology Nutritionist: Will address any nutritional and/or dietary concerns during the course of cancer treatment

Oncology Nurse Navigator: Will guide you through the cancer process and make sure you have all referrals and follow-up visits scheduled for the appropriate medical professionals during your journey

Primary Care Physician (and associated staff such as a Physician's Assistant or Nurse Practitioner): Will assist in monitoring other body systems that may have been affected by cancer and make referrals to other medical professionals as appropriate.

Phlebotomist: Will perform blood draws to accompany any tests that are requested by your medical team

Medical Technician: Will administer scans and tests as ordered by your medical team if specialized treatments or processes are required

Physical Therapist: Will address any physical deficits or functional decline through guided exercise during or after your treatment. Will also address cancer-related fatigue and endurance for physical activity.

Occupational Therapist: Will assist in addressing any deficits or decline in your ability to perform activities of daily living such as bathing, dressing, cooking, cleaning, driving

Speech Therapist: Will address any swallowing issues and/or speech and cognitive deficits in addition to "chemo-brain" or "chemo-fog" that can result as a side effect from chemotherapy and radiation treatments

Lymphedema Therapist: Will address lymphedema (swelling) and improper functioning of the lymphatic system that can result from cancer-related surgery, chemotherapy, and radiation.

Psychologist: Will address mental health concerns and provide you with coping mechanisms help you or your family members before, during, or after your treatment.

Genetic Counselor: Will help you and your family understand your inherited cancer risk as well as offer information about cancer screening, prevention, and treatment options and provide support.

Social Worker: Will assist in providing you with community resources as they relate to medical transportation, resources for financial concerns, community medical screenings, referrals for cancer support groups

<u>Home Health Care Nurse:</u> Will assist in ensuring proper medication administration at home as well as assist in managing any medical paraphernalia (foley catheters, drainage tubes, surgical wounds and associated dressings)

<u>Home Health Care Aide:</u> Will assist with household chores and daily grooming tasks if needed during or after your treatment

<u>Medical Specialists or Surgeons:</u> This is highly dependent upon the type of cancer diagnosed and how it has affected other organs and/or bodily systems. Examples of these professionals include neurologists, nephrologists, breast specialists, pulmonologists, ear/nose/throat specialists, radiologists, gynecologists, urologists, cardiologists, and pain management specialists; to name a few.

___Do not assume that your medical team will automatically refer you to the other professionals that are listed above. Do not be afraid to ask your physician to refer you to a professional if you feel that it is a service that you need or will benefit from (i.e. Physical Therapist).

___Be sure to inform your doctor and other members of your medical team of what your post-treatment goals are. What activities do you hope to return to doing? Do you plan to return to work? Do you plan to travel? Do you plan to return to your pre-diagnosis workout routine? This will help your medical team give you further guidance on expected time frames for return to these activities.

___Request a detailed treatment summary of all tests, procedures, treatments, and medications that you have had for your own records so that you are well informed about your cancer treatment course. This is also essential in the event that you change healthcare providers or change your place of residence and your new medical team asks you questions regarding your cancer history and care received.

Section 2: Financial Considerations

The absolute last thing a cancer patient should have to concern themselves with is how the cost of their medical treatment will be paid for. However, the reality is, it is a very important component among the many other considerations to contend with during such a trying time.

Consider the following:

___What your doctor's office will want to determine is the type of insurance you have; if any. In most instances, your doctor is not the one with whom you will address financial concerns. You will, in all likelihood, interact with the office manager or a member of the office finance staff to discuss what you need to understand about the costs associated with your treatment.

Keep in mind, they will only discuss the cost of the treatment they provide and/or the fees associated with office visits (such as co-payments, coinsurance payments, special medications, procedures, etc.) They are not prepared to discuss the costs for inpatient or outpatient hospital/clinic visits (procedures, tests, personnel, treatment) or supplies purchased/leased at pharmacies or medical supply companies (such as commode seats, oxygen equipment, first aid supplies) and the myriad of other items that could be necessary dependent upon your specific issues.

___It is also advisable to meet with a financial counselor to learn the out-of-pocket expenses for all of your treatment options, money matters and/or help with insurance benefit claims.

Patients That Have Insurance Coverage:

___Check on your health insurance coverage by having a conversation with your insurance company(s). Ensure that you understand precisely:

___What medical coverage you have.

___Whether you have met any or all of your obligations (annual deductible, maximum out-of-pocket.)

___What payment would be due (if any) at the time of each office visit.

___What payment (if any) would be due at the time of hospitalization.

___What to expect when treatment expenses are submitted for payment.

___What pre-authorization for services is required, if any

___Coverage for surgical procedures

___Coverage for prescription medications, both brand-name and generic

___What you need to consider should the need arise for treatment by specialists (physicians aside from your Primary Care Physician (PCP) and what coverage you have for those situations.

___Aside from office visits, hospitalization and medication coverage, inquire as to coverage for services such as Physical Therapy or other rehabilitation therapy services such as Occupational Therapy and Speech therapy in settings of home health, inpatient rehabilitation facility, and an outpatient rehabilitation facility or clinic.

___Home Health Care Services: Nursing, Home Health Aides

___Hospice Services: Both inpatient and outpatient settings

___Palliative Care Services

___Coverage for supplies and durable medical equipment (DME) to be obtained if ordering from medical supply companies, such as:

• Wound care supplies

• First Aid Supplies

• Assistive devices and other apparatus (commode seats, walkers, canes, wheelchairs, hospital beds, compression garments, hoyer lifts, compression pumps, oxygen tanks/ concentrators, incontinence products, wigs, breast prostheses, catheter bottles, colostomy paraphernalia and many other items.)

___Which medical supply or durable medical equipment (DME) companies can be utilized.

___Should counseling be recommended by your physician, are the fees covered?

___Coverage for inpatient rehabilitation stays if needed to help you improve your physical functioning if recommended by your medical team during the course of your treatment.

When discussing impending financial costs with the physician's office, make certain to have the following items available:

___The name of and member identification number for your primary insurance company. Should you have a member identification card, all of the pertinent information would be included on it, so that the office personnel will want to review it and obtain whatever is necessary.

___The name of and member identification number for any secondary insurance that you may have. Again, have all pertinent information ready to provide the office personnel.

___Another purpose for verification of your insurance coverage would be to ensure that your medical provider is within the insurance company's network.

This is something that you can verify yourself via the membership documentation received from the insurance company(s) upon sign-up. You can also check the insurance company's website or call the customer service number (usually printed on the member's identification card.)

If your insurance provider is not 'in network,' you will most likely have only two options:

- To remain with the out-of-network provider and be considered 'self-pay.' (Self-pay is discussed in the following section.)

- To request a referral to another physician, locate one on your own, or ask your insurance company for referral assistance.

Patients That Do Not Have Insurance Coverage:

___If you do not have insurance (or you have insurance, but the physician is out-of-network), you will be considered 'self-pay.' Although this will seem harsh, many medical practices will not treat patients who do not have some form of insurance. This is totally at the discretion of the individual physician. Some health care providers accept patients who will be responsible for payment of their own medical costs. Should your physician accept self-pay patients, make certain that you have a thorough discussion with the office personnel regarding:

___What the anticipated charges will be

___What the self-pay requirements are o When payments are required

___What forms of payment are accepted (cash, checks (personal or certified funds), credit cards, debit cards, automatic deduction)

___What payment plans are available if applicable

___If you are currently employed, it is important that you know what benefits your employer allows in regards to paid-time-off (PTO), vacation time, sick leave, and Family Medical Leave of Absence (FMLA) requirements.

___You should also inquire if your employer provides short-term disability and long-term disability benefits or if free counseling services are offered. You also also know what medical documentation is required, if any, for you to provide to your employer to receive such benefits.

Additional Resources:

There are agencies, foundations and organizations that offer financial help. The key is finding them and then determining what the qualifications are for applying and assistance consideration.

For example:

There is availability through Medicaid; the Women's Breast Cancer Program. Qualifications include the following:

- A confirmed diagnosis of breast cancer. A full copy of your medical records detailing the diagnosis must be submitted.

- You cannot presently have any form of insurance coverage. This will be verified by the agency.

- You cannot exceed certain income limits.

- The program is not administered via the Social Security office. You would need to contact the local Medicaid office, usually listed under the county offices where you reside.

The Elements Of Cancer Survivorship

___Inquire at your primary care physician's office, in addition to your oncologist's office for agencies, foundations or organizations that they may be aware of that offer cancer-care assistance and support. In addition, research online for groups that specialize in cancer awareness, advocacy and assistance. There are literally hundreds of them available; far too many to list here.

The Elements Of Cancer Survivorship

Section 3: Support And Advocacy

We stressed how the diagnosis of cancer affects not only the body, but the mind, will, and emotions as well. While it may seem cliché, one of the greatest needs during the cancer process is for you to have impactful interaction with others; particularly other cancer survivors. There are many ways by which you can gain the support of others who care and can empathize with your situation.

Sympathy is one thing, which merely means that someone feels sorry for your plight and issues but cannot really understand what it is like to live with what is often seen as a death sentence. Empathy is completely different! When someone empathizes with you, they can feel what you feel, understand your fears, and not ridicule your anger, frustration, feelings of hopelessness and uncertainty and the fact that you might have good days and bad days emotionally. **DO NOT OVERLOOK OR UNDERESTIMATE THE IMPORTANCE OF THIS ESSENTIAL ASPECT OF THE PROCESS!**

Set your mind to getting support for yourself and for being an advocate! You need practical help at home and you need to get involved with the advocacy community. Support is so important during those 'bad days.' Helping others during their bad days will help strengthen you as well. Studies have proven that seeking support during cancer treatment can actually help boost the effectiveness of your treatment and even improve the outcome! Fortunately, there are various ways by which you can obtain the support. No one way works for everyone.

Here are some of the methods available to choose from:

<u>Face-to-Face Support Groups:</u> These are usually led by a person trained to keep control of the conversation so that it is productive, positive and informative. While the eye contact, conversa-

tional setting is best for some, it can be unnerving for others who are uncomfortable in talking about their condition, personal life and their innermost feelings among perfect strangers. It also may not be the right setting if a person is seeking information for their particular type and stage of cancer and might not want to listen to stories about other types of cancer. Ask your oncologist or a social worker for information about local support groups. You might also call the local hospitals to inquire as to whether they have such a group for cancer patients. Also, research online the type of cancer you are under treatment for and look for support group information.

Online Help: Unlike in-person groups that meet at specific times, online support groups offer support when you want or need it. Someone would be available at any hour of the day or night to answer your post. Message boards and forums also enable you to connect with people using your therapy. A good way to locate an online group is to go to the website for the therapy/medical treatment that you are using, (i.e. Receiving chemotherapy? Search for the website for the type of chemo medication that you are using. Also, you can search for the type of cancer you are diagnosed with, which may also have an online group available for you to join.)

Telephone or Email Support Programs: These endeavors are usually manned by other cancer survivors who have been trained to mentor, encourage and support you. Volunteers are matched as closely as possible to your request. Connecting with someone else is invaluable when they have been matched to your comfort level in regard to gender, age, are parents with small children, length of cancer treatment, length of remission, same treatment as you are receiving, and other particulars that you have stipulated. Search for these types of programs in the same way you would search for the online help group as mentioned above.

Medical Advice: Talk with your doctor when you need advice, input or have concerns. In addition, you can talk with a nurse at your insurance company should this option be available to you. Another thought would be to request a referral from your doctor or the nurse to another physician or a treatment center in your area to get a second opinion.

<u>Support Your Peers:</u> A good place to start is to get involved with organizations equipped to provide the help you need and will enable you to help others. Ask how you can get involved. Maybe you can answer support telephone lines, be a mentor for another individual that share's your cancer diagnosis, or help with in-person support groups or by providing online support.

<u>Personal Advocacy:</u> Advocacy is about standing up and being a voice for something you feel strongly about. You are promoting change because you are unhappy with the status quo and want to take a stand for issues that you are passionate about. When it comes to cancer, there are many aspects that you may feel need to change, such as insurance regulations or cancer research funding by the government. Think about your own journey and those aspects that were troublesome or difficult for you. That may help you to know what you may want to advocate for.

<u>Patient Advocacy:</u> In this capacity, you would be providing support for individuals or groups of people. There are lots of ways to get involved, such as working with local hospitals to ensure cancer patients are receiving the care, treatment and support that they need. You could work with researchers who are doing clinical trials, ensuring they are recruiting participants appropriately and that the patients have an opportunity to express their point of view. Other opportunities may exist to serve on government grant committees involved with providing funding.

Section 4: The Power Of Hope

Hope: (According to Webster's New World Dictionary, Fourth Edition) means:

1. A feeling that what is wanted will happen; desire accompanied by expectation.

2. A person or thing on which one may base some hope.

Too many patients are navigating the uncertain, churning waters of cancer without a key ingredient: **HOPE!** Read the definition of hope over and over to yourself and let it sink in, then ask yourself if you truly have the ingredient of hope or is it sincerely missing from your life and journey.

True enough, cancer patients must interact with the healthcare professionals, who test us, diagnose us, prescribe for us, operate on us, administer treatment for us, pronounce our potential to live a life in remission, or our probability to succumb to the ravages of cancer while heading to the inevitable. They are doing their job in telling us what their findings are. At least we are not in the previous times when it was thought best not to tell patients the truth about their condition, especially if the anticipated outcome was that they would not get better. That thought affords little comfort when it is you to whom a dire diagnosis is being given.

So what is the answer? If the definition for hope is not firmly entrenched within you, there are two choices. You can either let despair and self-pity sweep over you in great mounting waves until the very effort of getting out of bed each day becomes more than you can manage, or you can take hold of hope, gain a confident expectation, and become the survivor that is possible if you can but believe.

Many doctors can tell of situations where everything indicated the patient would not recover, but can attest how the power of positive thinking, positive speaking and a positive expectation absolutely turned the tide and aided in the patient's recovery. Constantly dwelling on how bad things are or having a continual "why me" attitude will only defeat you. Expect the best in hope (a confident expectation) and you will see the best come forth (the expectation can actually become real.)

How to stay hopeful:

___Realize that even in the worst of times, you can strive to make life the best it can be.

___Hoping for the best will mobilize you to make health-promoting steps that improve your chances to experience the desired outcome.

___Stay away from focusing on statistics. This is a hard one. Daily, it seems that there is constant information regarding cancer and how many "do not make it." Hearing all the negativity about cancer can definitely rob you of hope.

___Stay active and involved in your overall treatment process. Try to maintain your normal daily routine and activities as much as possible so that it encourages and motivates you to return to your pre-cancer state of functioning.

___Limit the amount of Google research that you do to only what is needful for the answers you require for your care. Do not spend time reading the woe is me, negative input from despairing cancer patients.

___ Do not give statistics and other patients experiences and fears power over you. Stay focused on the positive! They are not you and you are not them! Their experience does not have to be your experience, nor their outcomes your outcome!

___Embrace life! You are still here! You are vital. To keep hope from fading away, you must take responsibility for yourself. Daily, you must take steps to energize your hope. Instead of listening to the negativity of others, focus on the cancer success stories of others. Get involved with helping others going through this cancer journey. Read uplifting and inspirational sayings. Listen to positive, uplifting music. Recite uplifting prayers.

___Do not be afraid to let people around you know how you are feeling and how they can help support you through the process. Oftentimes, loved ones are also afraid and overwhelmed and want to help you as much as possible, but are unsure of what to do or what to say. Only you know what your needs are. You owe it to yourself to let others know what is and isn't helpful to you during your journey.

___Subscribe to cancer magazines, journals, or newsletters that are filled with positive and informative content.

___Purpose not to let cancer steal your life; literally or figuratively. You must accept a new normal, and many things will have to be done differently, but you can still control how you think.

___Allow a very small momentary pity party, but know that your thoughts, words and actions can influence how you physically feel. Refuse to allow a negative mindset to stay. Shift your mood.

___Consider journaling or keeping a diary. Get those negative feelings out! Allow the positive feelings in! Document how you feel during the entire process. Talk an attitude of gratitude. Remember, it could always be worse!

___Most of all ---NEVER GIVE UP!

Resources

- What is Survivorship? American Society of Clinical Oncology (ASCO). Accessed online at https://www.cancer.net/survivorship/what-survivorship

- National Cancer Insitiute Division of Cancer Control and Population Sciences.

- Accessed online at https://cancercontrol.cancer.gov/ocs/statistics/statistics.html

- Cancer Treatment and Survivorship Facts and Figures by The American Cancer Society. Accessed online at https://www.cancer.org/content/dam/cancer-org/research/cancer-facts-andstatistics/cancer-treatment-and-survivorship-facts-and-figures/cancer-treatmentand-survivorship-facts-and-figures-2016-2017.pdf

- Healthmonitor Guide to Chemotherapy/True Inspiration (Jennifer Martinez)

- Coping With Cancer, March/April 2018/Moving Forward as a Lung Cancer Survivor

- Webster's New World Dictionary, Fourth Edition

About The Authors

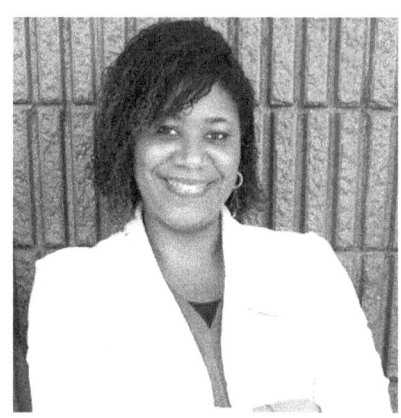

Dr. Crystal A. Champion

White Plains, Georgia native Dr. Crystal A. Champion, PT, DPT, CLT, Cert. DN, is a Physical Therapist and a Certified Lymphedema Therapist. Upon graduating from Greene-Taliaferro Comprehensive High School in Greensboro, Georgia in 2000 as Valedictorian, Dr. Champion attended Georgia College & State University in Milledgeville, Georgia where she graduated Cum Laude and obtained a Bachelor of Science Degree in Health Education with a Concentration in Exercise Science in 2004. She was also initiated into Alpha Kappa Alpha Sorority, Inc in which she remains an active member in the Upsilon Alpha Omega Chapter in Gwinnett County, Georgia. Dr. Champion attended the Medical College of Georgia where she obtained a Master of Physical Therapy degree in 2006 and a Doctor of Physical Therapy Degree in 2008.

Dr. Champion has served on various committees to include the Cancer Committee, Oncology Continuous Quality Improvement Team, Unit Practice Council, and the Palliative Care Team. She has also served as a host committee member for an Atlanta signature fundraiser, Jeffrey Fashion Cares, which supports Susan G. Komen Atlanta and the Atlanta AIDS Fund. In her career, she has received accolades to include the Innovators Award for Quality/Patient Safety, a Clinical Excellence Award, and was nominated for the American Health Council Best In Patient Care Award. She is also an American Physical Therapy Association Credentialed Clinical Instructor in which she facilitates clinical experiences for students in Doctor of Physical Therapy programs. Dr. Champion has a special interest in oncology rehabilitation and was instrumental in developing the oncology rehabilitation program as well as the outpatient lymphedema treatment program for Emory Johns Creek Hospital. She obtained her certification as a Lymphedema Therapist from the Academy of Lymphatic Studies and recently completed her certifications in Advanced Lymphedema Management as well as Dry Needling. She also lectures to breast surgery fellows at Winship Cancer Institute of Emory and participates in various community events to spread awareness about cancer survivorship.

Dr. Champion has had family and friends that have been affected by cancer and have endured horrible sideeffects, leading to decline in physical functioning and a poor quality of life. Her passion for providing quality care for patients who require cancer rehabilitation and lymphedema therapy led her to start her own practice, Eminence Physical Therapy, LLC. Also, in her experience as a healthcare practitioner, she saw the need to serve cancer patients on a larger scale and encourage patients take a more holistic approach to restoring their psychological well-being, physical functioning, and quality of life as often the physical, psychological, spiritual, and emotional impairments resulting from cancer treatment are often not addressed or are improperly addressed.

This led her to establish Champions Can! Foundation for Cancer Wellness, Inc., a 501 (c)(3) nonprofit organization that promotes and advocates for cancer survivorship. Dr. Champion has gained more awareness surrounding the gaps in cancer education as well as the limited focus on cancer survivorship once cancer treatment has been completed. Her organization hopes to be the leader in the promotion of cancer survivorship.

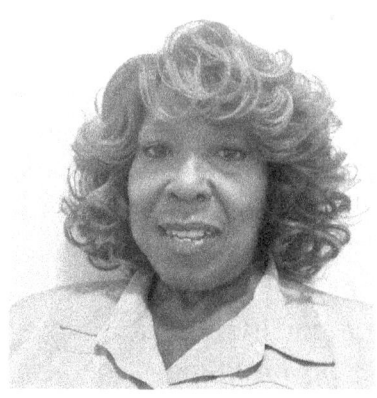

Marcia D. Dupree

Pastor Marcia D. DuPree has a strong background in teaching and training, having spent 24 years employed by a major corporation as a trainer/teacher, course developer and a staff manager. She is also a Life Member of the National Council of Negro Women. In 1993 she began the Sisters in Christ women's ministry which met monthly in her home. In 1996, she sensed that it was time to step out and fulfill a dream that had been in her heart for many years.

She moved to Tulsa, Oklahoma to attend RHEMA Bible Training College, graduating in 1998. In 1999, she and her husband started Enriching Your World Family Church in Atlanta, GA, which in 2004, was relocated to Jonesboro, a suburb of Atlanta. Pastor Marcy, as she was known to her congregants, has been an invited speaker and teacher at women's retreats, church services, and Bible schools. She has also traveled to the Philippines and Indonesia, ministering the gospel. Her philosophy is to preach and teach with "accuracy, clarity and simplicity, so they that hear may understand," and thereby be equipped to put into practice her shared truths and insights. In January of 2017, Marcia experienced one of her greatest tests of courage and fortitude, in that she was diagnosed with metastatic breast cancer. While her faith has stood her in good stead and provided the grounding needed to withstand the trials experienced when coping with such a serious illness, she recognized the difficulties patients encounter when facing the initial diagnosis of cancer and how ill equipped most patients are. What's the next step when hearing that dreaded diagnosis? What questions should be asked? What should I expect of the medical/surgical team?

What major lifestyle changes will I encounter? The uncertainties can seem daunting and insurmountable. Marcia had also found that she lacked a lot of the information and guidance needed at the onset of the cancer journey. Her heart for helping, supporting and teaching others prompted Marcia to become a board member and Vice President of Champions Can! Foundation for Cancer Wellness, Inc. and to take on the task of compiling this booklet. The purpose is to equip those in the initial throes of a cancer diagnosis or those well along the treatment trail to be enlightened with insights that can help them be advocates for their own wellness.

Champions Can! Foundation for Cancer Wellness, Inc.

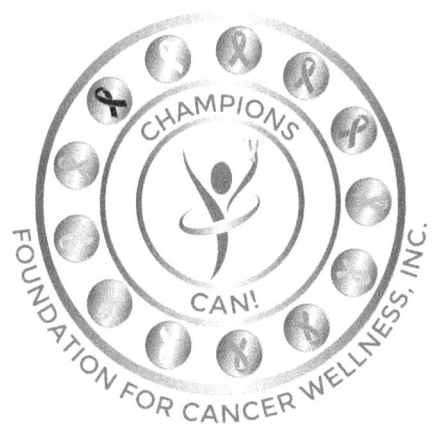

"Unite, Strive, Educate, Survive!"

Mission Statement:

Champions Can! Foundation for Cancer Wellness, Inc. is a nonprofit 501(c)(3) organization that advocates for cancer survivorship by striving to provide services to unite, support and educate individuals before, during, and after their course of cancer treatment with the goal of promoting cancer survivorship and improving quality of life, regardless of the cancer diagnosis.

Purpose:

Champions Can! Foundation for Cancer Wellness, Inc. offers a comprehensive cancer wellness program with a holistic approach that will provide and achieve the following:

- Restoration of physical functioning through the promotion of physical fitness and physical activity

- Restoration of psychological and spiritual well-being through counseling, chaplaincy, energy healing, meditation, and other appropriate methods

- Promotion of healthy eating and nutritional counseling to aid in physical healing

- Coordination and referral of other community resources per individual need

- Community education regarding cancer care, post-cancer care, cancer survivorship, and cancer recovery

- Improvement of self-esteem through the enhancement of physical appearance and referral to appropriate resources

- Support of cancer survivors and their families and/or caregivers through the recovery process

- Evidence-based research and backing for services that are offered

Contact:

Website: www.facebook.com/championscan

Email: championscanfoundation@gmail.com